ALONG THE CONTINUUM OF CARE

ALONG THE CONTINUUM OF CARE

WHAT EVERY CASE MANAGER MUST KNOW . . .

PAULINE SANDERS RN, MBA, CCM

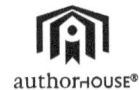

authorHOUSE®

AuthorHouse™
1663 Liberty Drive
Bloomington, IN 47403
www.authorhouse.com
Phone: 1-800-839-8640

Published by AuthorHouse   05/14/2013

ISBN: 978-1-4817-4548-2 (sc)
ISBN: 978-1-4817-4547-5 (e)

Library of Congress Control Number: 2013907244

Any people depicted in stock imagery provided by Thinkstock are models, and such images are being used for illustrative purposes only.
Certain stock imagery © Thinkstock.

This book is printed on acid-free paper.

Because of the dynamic nature of the Internet, any web addresses or links contained in this book may have changed since publication and may no longer be valid. The views expressed in this work are solely those of the author and do not necessarily reflect the views of the publisher, and the publisher hereby disclaims any responsibility for them.

DEDICATION

This book is dedicated to my Mom and Dad who gave me a great start in life and to my two wonderful sons, Dale and Josh, who have expanded my experiences in life.

ACKNOWLEDGMENTS

I want to express the highest gratitude for the people who have helped me to meet the challenges to write this book. Special thanks goes out to Georgette "Gigi" Ligons, my business manager, from *Braylen James Business Solutions* who has cheered me on and supported me in sharing my passion about case management with the health care world. From the bottom of my heart, I want to thank my executive coach and mentor, Mark Susnow, Esq., of *Inspire Possibility* for moving me to this project, moving me through my commitments and being there to keep me on track when procrastination started. I could not have done this without you. Thank You.

THE CHANGING PARADIGM
OF CASE MANAGEMENT

"Either you're an agent of change, or you're destined to become a victim of change. You simply can't survive over the long term if you insist on standing still."

- Norm Brodsky, entrepreneur

The urgent need to improve health outcomes is resulting in moment-to-moment changes in the world of case management. This means that "agent of change" and "resource connector" must now be added to the case manager's multiple roles.

Ready or not, the future has arrived. Case managers find themselves being called to be more flexible and adaptable than ever before. They must approach their work with open minds and innovative ideas.

When moving patients along the continuum of care, many things go when they meet the patient's needs in an acceptable manner, even if it goes against the grain of what was done in the past.

Case managers have only one goal and that is to ensure their care plans provides quality care for their patients at a reasonable cost to the health care systems.

This book is designed to help healthcare professionals understand effective case management and to meet the challenges of this exciting and essential profession. In the coming chapters there will be details on the tools and ideas case managers will need to better equip themselves to negotiate through this brave new world of health care. At the same time, there will be a continuing focus on the need for case managers to handle themselves and their patients with competency and integrity.

This book is based on the concept that to succeed in case management, it is essential for business logic to be applied to all decisions. As a result, the focus is not just on theory and standards of excellence in practice, but also on essential skills like critical thinking, streams of revenue for health care providers, the high costs of avoidable days of care, and the tools needed to negotiate one's way along the continuum of care.

Based on years of practice in the field, the author will also offer advice about dealing with all the components of the health care system including difficult patients, families and physicians. The components of the case manager's toolkit will be defined, a bank of resources outlined, and the importance of professionalism stressed in every step of the process.

In order to handle each patient along the continuum of care, case managers must be able to determine where the patient came from and have a projection of where his/her final destination will be. The patient may come from home and return home but may transition to several interim destinations for skilled services or to have rehabilitation before returning home.

Effective case managers are able to decrease the degree of fragmentation by carefully helping the multidisciplinary team plan for short term and long term goals. If the initial case manager needs to hand off the patient to another case manager along the continuum, a well-established plan will decrease chaos and make the transition an effective one to ensure that the patient is safe.

The modern case manager must be able to envision what the global picture looks like for each and every patient for whom he or she provides care coordination.

This book is designed to enhance understanding of the expectations of a case manager in most areas that are encountered along the care continuum. For those already working as a case manager, this will be an excellent refresher. For chief executive officers, physicians and those in senior leadership roles, it will be a simple clarification of their roles in supporting and assisting case managers.

For nurses, social workers, and health care workers who are expecting to transition into case management, or for those who have the desire to pursue this career, this will be a valuable reference book.

Health care case management is defined as moving the patient along the continuum of care to ensure they are receiving quality care while attempting to contain health care costs. This is accomplished by monitoring the patient's health status to be certain they are at the appropriate level on the continuum. In the first chapter, "The Continuum of Care" will be defined and discussed.

Case management involves the multidisciplinary health care teams' collaboration to establish the optimum plan of care with the patient and the family.

The work case managers do has never been more crucial to the health care industry. Case management practices are reducing the amount of inappropriate dollars that are being used to keep patients in higher levels of care when their care can safely be moved to the next lower level.

Although there are many definitions for the role of the case manager, the essential components all lead to one common goal and destination. Their goal is to maintain quality care to the patient and to perform that quality care in an appropriate setting. The destination is to have used the allotted resources wisely to improve patient satisfaction, patient healing, and patient dignity, while reducing costs to the health care industry.

As the case management profession moves forward, it is important to initially consider the key components of the health care continuum.

CHAPTER ONE

THE CONTINUUM OF CARE

"Diagnosis is not the end, but the beginning of practice."

- Martin H. Fischer

A case manager is often said to be managing a patient "along the continuum of care." This means managing a patient's care in multiple settings from the beginning of an illness until the patient is no longer ill and no longer under a medical regime.

For patients who are terminal or have chronic illnesses, the continuum of care may become a recurring cycle until the end of life.

Case managers, along with the health care team, identify and address medical needs, financial needs, psychological needs, family needs, and resource needs at each level to ensure a smooth transition from one level to the next.

The intent of an effective case manager is to anticipate a patient's needs prior to moving him/her to the next level. Through proper set up and family preparation, the necessary resources are in place when the patient is ready to transition from hospital to skilled nursing, skilled rehabilitation, home health, or to home.

In the case of a patient who is chronically ill, the transition would be from the acute care, to perhaps a skilled setting, and then back home with the community clinic, doctor's office, or medical home model to support the patient as needed. The ideal model is to have a trained case manager available as a contact for care coordination in the community and at the home to proactively promote compliance with the plan of care. This helps prevent unnecessary readmissions to the hospital.

In the United States, the current health care model supports the case management process in every health care setting. Case managers in the hospitals can coordinate care for the patient and the family prior to discharge by knowing the plan of care and effectively performing discharge planning evaluations.

Case managers can and should communicate with other case managers along the continuum of care to prepare for the patient's seamless transitions from the hospital to the final discharge disposition.

In the case of a patient who is on palliative care, end of life, and hospice care, the case managers will be the pivotal support for the patient and the family at the end of life process.

As a patient moves along the continuum of care, case managers need to be aware of the business of health care while simultaneously managing the needs of the patient. A huge challenge is to be aware of the high cost of what are called "avoidable days."

When patients are in the hospital, skilled facilities, or acute rehabilitation centers without meeting the established criteria to be in that setting, the institution is losing money unnecessarily. These are avoidable days. Many facilities track avoidable days to routinely review the data and determine if there are trends and to improve the discharge process if there are uniform system issues.

One example of avoidable days is a patient who is difficult to place in a skilled rehabilitation due to numerous co-morbidities that would require more resources than the desired facility can adequately provide in order for the patient to receive optimum care.

Another example of avoidable days is a new orthopedic surgeon who is well known for allowing his/her patients to remain in the hospital past their stabilization period for discharge solely because the patient wants to stay one more day.

Avoidable days can quickly add up to millions of dollars in annual loss revenues for an institution. The case manager is one of the key members of the health care team who should be anticipating the needs of the patients on his/her caseload and having a collaborative conversation with the physician about the best approach to take with potential problems.

Case managers who will be working along the continuum of care will find themselves based either in health care settings or working with various agencies and organizations that provide health care.

Many of the settings encountered along the continuum of care are:

Ambulatory Care—This setting is synonymous with community clinics and sometimes doctors' offices depending on the care provided in these settings. The care could be similar. However, there may be specialties and subspecialty clinics within the larger ambulatory care centers.

Community Clinics—Many community-based case managers may work with specific populations such as HIV, diabetes, chronic heart diseases, and the frail elderly. These populations could benefit from a team case management approach which could involve a nurse and/ or a medical social worker. The community clinic patients may have many social and family issues that will need to be addressed. The case manager in this role attempts to keep the patients and their families compliant with the medical plan of care.

Home Health—The home care case manager's role greatly assists the health care industry in cutting high costs that are endured for unnecessary stays in the hospital, skilled nursing, and/or rehabilitation facilities. It has been proven that most patients would like to receive care in their own home and many family members want to have their loved ones at home. The demand with home care case management will only increase with the aging population and the implementation of health care reform. The family may be required to take on a larger role in helping with the patient's care when they remain in the home. The goals of home care are to decrease health care costs by keeping patients from being admitted to higher levels of care, monitor the patients to ensure compliance with the plan of care, improve the quality of care, and work with the case managers along the continuum of care to aid the patient in having a seamless transition from one place to the next.

Hospital—This is the acute care setting. The facility may be a general hospital which includes an emergency room, critical care, intensive care, medical units, surgical units, obstetrical units, pediatrics, and newborn nurseries. There are many hospitals that are facilities which may not include all of the services as that of a general hospital.

Hospice—The hospice case manager is the primary person to coordinate care for the patient and the family during the end of life process. The role of the case manager is to make sure the patient receives adequate comfort care during their terminal illness, ensure that the family needs are met, and assist with bereavement services. Most hospice cases are managed in the patient's home but the patient may also be institutionalized in the hospital or skilled nursing facility.

Medical Home—The medical home is a relatively new model that has come into place with health care reform. Medical homes are defined as regular health care providers that offer timely, well-organized care and enhanced access. The case manager in this model will again be the pivotal person to coordinate the care with the physician and the health care team to ensure continuity of care. The physician will be the primary person directing the care but the case manager will be the person who coordinates and establishes that the right personnel is providing the care which is being directed by the physician.

This model is still in the development phase, but there is a high degree of interest in the medical home model by federal, state and local government. This model could easily become the referral program for the future of health care.

Skilled Nursing Facility—The skilled nursing facility case manager manages the patient usually for a short period of time. Patients mostly come from the hospital setting to continue the healing process before being discharged home. The skilled nursing case manager can seem to be somewhat sandwiched between hospital case managers and the community case managers. The case manager should continue a smooth plan of care, along with the expectations of the multidisciplinary team, to assist the patient and their family to get home. The skilled case manager must anticipate the home needs and discuss discharge plans with the home health, community case manager, or the case manager at the medical home.

Outside of these health care settings, case managers specialize in working in many other areas along the continuum of care. These include acute rehabilitation, chronic disease management, the homeless, pediatrics, or school nursing. Listed below is a summary of the role of case managers in these various settings:

Acute Rehabilitation—The rehabilitation case manager works with the patient, family, and multidisciplinary team to establish short-term and long-term goals to restore a handicapped individual to his/her fullest physical, mental, social, vocational, and economic capabilities. The rehabilitation case manager should know that a patient in acute rehab must be able to participate in therapy at a minimum of three hours a day.

Chronic Disease Management—Case management of the chronically ill patient has proven to be a positive movement for all involved, including the patient, their families, and the providers. The case managers for this group of patients play a key role in building relationships, assisting the patient in understanding and complying with the plan of care that is designed for them specifically. Case managing the chronically ill patient in the outpatient setting has proven to decrease readmissions in the acute care hospital.

Homeless—The case manager for the homeless may be managing them as a result of a recent discharge from the hospital or as one of the chronically ill patients who are being managed in the community clinics under specific programs such as the HIV program.

Pediatrics/Children—The pediatric case manager must involve a multidisciplinary team to determine the plan of care for children.

This category of case management will be discussed in more detail in Chapter Seven.

School Nursing—The school nurse or case manager is an important role that is not widely talked about. Most public school districts employ nurses, social workers, and/or health care case workers to assist with the management of children who have illnesses and chronic diseases. Some large school districts may employ many nurses or case managers to handle medical service programs. The federal government in the United States also mandates the early, periodic screening, diagnosis and treatment plans for children with disabilities. The multidisciplinary team should include the case manager, the parents, and the primary care physician or speciality physician. The case manager ensures that each child's plan supports the immunizations, vision and hearing screening, and preventive wellness child visits.

Additionally, other case managers will work with specific agencies, departments and organizations involved along the continuum of care. Some of these include the Department of Justice, insurance companies, or Worker's Compensation.

Department of Justice—Some department of law enforcement facilities employ case workers to manage the plan of care for individuals who are incarcerated and have chronic illnesses. This could include adults as well as juveniles.

Insurance Companies—The case manager who works for the insurance company may be assigned to a variety of different roles. The case manager may handle the claims, pre certifications, telephonic case management for patients in the hospitals, skilled facilities, or many other duties. Insurance based case management can be very complex. The case manager is expected to know the state regulations for the coverage plan to ensure that benefits are coordinated correctly.

Worker's Compensation—The Worker's Compensation case manager manages a caseload of workers who have been injured on the job and who are now on temporary leave or may eventually be put on permanent disability. Many organizations employ case workers to manage injured workers' cases. The case manager's role in workers compensation cases involve monitoring, evaluating, and reporting outcomes to the employer. The case manager may provide limited assistance in referring the injured worker and his family to appropriate providers and agencies that are approved by the insurance company to handle the claims for the employer. The case worker may follow the injured worker who has suffered catastrophic injuries such as head injuries, spinal cord injuries, severe burns, amputations, and major organ and other severe damages.

To serve such a wide variety of positions along the health care continuum, the successful case manager will need a variety of tools and resources. In the next chapter, the essentials of the toolkit will be unveiled.

Suggested additional reading: "Standards of Practice for Case Management" (revised 2010), the voluntary practice guidelines for the case management industry published by the Case Management Society of America (http://www.cmsa.org/Individual/MemberToolkit/ StandardsofPractice/tabid/69/Default.aspx). Available electronically for download on the CMSA site or in printed copy.

CHAPTER TWO

THE CASE MANAGER'S TOOLKIT

"My own experience is to use the tools that are out there. Use the digital world. But never lose sight of the need to reach out and talk to other people who don't share your view. Listen to them and see if you can find a way to compromise."

- Colin Powell

We have learned what case managers do in their various roles and details in some of the settings along the continuum of care. We are aware of the high cost of avoidable days and the importance of moving patients into appropriate settings.

One big question looms: How do case managers determine if a patient meets the criteria for their current treatment setting?

The effective case manager builds up a toolkit that can be applied to every individual situation to assist them in determining which patients should remain where they are, and which should be moved to another setting.

This toolkit includes such software programs as InterQual and/or Milliman Guidelines, medical necessity criteria, clinical education, and expert resources. Some organizations have created their own homegrown software tools to accommodate the guidelines for measuring whether or not the patient is at the appropriate level of care.

Another essential tool, medical record documentation, will be dealt with in a separate chapter. Documentation is particularly vital because it must support the set criteria in order for the health care facility to receive the reimbursement to which it is entitled.

It is recommended that health care case managers have three to five years of experience in the medical field as a nurse, social worker, or health care worker to be able to fully understand and function as preferred case managers. If one is entering the field of case management without that level of experience, one is encouraged to identify a role model or mentor who can assist him/her for the first six to twelve months to help one to function more confidently.

Case managers use medical necessity criteria to determine the appropriateness of a patient's care. Patients must meet established criteria to justify the charges that will be reimbursed by insurance companies.

The insurance companies may include government payers such as Medicare, Medicaid, Medi-Cal (California), or private insurance such as Blue Cross, Blue Shield, AETNA, etc. Patients may also pay for health care privately.

One of the commercial medical necessity tools in the health care market is InterQual Medical Necessity Criteria. It is widely used in the health care industry to determine if patients are meeting the criteria to be admitted to an acute care hospital. It is based on two concepts: the severity of illness and the intensity of service. Once a patient meets the criteria to be admitted, the tool is then used to determine if the daily stay in the hospital is justified.

Interqual is a product that is produced by the McKesson Corporation and they offer in depth training to organizations that buy their products. Hospitals must purchase a license to use this software in their facilities.

Another commercial medical necessity tools used in the health care market is Milliman Guidelines Medical Necessity Criteria. These guidelines, which have been around since the early 1980s and have been continuously updated, tend to use critical pathway guidance in which certain expectations are aligned with daily progress.

Listed is an example of Milliman's Guidelines: A certain diagnosis is expected to keep a patient in the hospital for four days. Day 1 would set specific goals; Day 2's goals would be set with the expectation that the patient progressed, and Day 3 and Day 4 likewise. The patient's goal is to be ready for discharge on Day 4.

Milliman guidelines were developed for providers to have guidance on treating common conditions that had few to no complications. Another example would be that of an elective surgery in an otherwise healthy person. Case management using these guidelines also benchmarks a patient's progress appropriately along the correct continuum of care.

There are other less popular tools in the market that are used by case managers to establish the appropriate admissions criteria and continued stay criteria, along with guidelines for appropriate discharge. As mentioned previously, some organizations have created their own home grown software.

Outside of the referenced software tools, case managers also have access to physician advisors who have oversight for the case management function from a medical standpoint. Physician advisors or the medical directors of case management can further justify the medical necessity and appropriateness for patients to be at the selected level of care along the continuum. The physician responsible for the patient's care has to document the pertinent plan of care for communication and reimbursement purposes. Patients must meet the established criteria to justify the charges that will be reimbursed by the insurance companies.

At this time there is no mandated use of any one method to establish medical necessity. Case managers must combine their use of effective tools with their clinical education, experience and skills in the medical field to accurately determine medical necessity.

Case managers must be conscious of their roles as "resource connectors." They are the key people to assist all levels of staff in the acute care hospital as well as along the entire continuum of care.

The case manager connects people with resources in the facilities, community and home.

An effective case manager should become familiar with the names and contact information of available resources and be able to impart these resources to the patients and their families. The compiled network for the case manager includes people, organizations, services, professional references, community references, or national references, as well as international references to provide referrals when planning care coordination.

As the case manager builds up a resource kit, it is also important to learn more about the financial side of health care and how it works. Financial aspects of health care will be addressed in the next chapter.

Take the time now to become familiar with medical necessity and charting guidelines using both InterQual and Milliman guidelines. Additional information is available on page 53-54 of The Case Manager's Training Manual by David W. Plocher and Patricia L. Metzger: (http://books. google.com/books/about/The_Case_Manager_s_Training_Manual. html?id=uZgrzk5Y4MAC)

CHAPTER THREE

WHAT CASE MANAGERS NEED TO KNOW ABOUT HEALTH CARE FINANCES

"Economy does not lie in sparing money, but in spending it wisely."

- Thomas Huxley

Case managers need to understand from the start that health care is a business. They must learn how to integrate business concepts into health care practices and maximize a win-win outcome for the patient and the health care community. Case managers face daily challenges with the process of providing quality care and integration of cost saving measures. The challenge is best managed when everyone involved, including the executive leadership team, understands and supports the integration through constant awareness of the case management process.

Traditionally, health care institutions found it difficult to view themselves as business entities since they were in the industry to help and heal the sick. As a result, over the past three to four decades, health care has become America's highest gross domestic product.

To balance economies in health care, people in the health professions have had to do a mental mind shift to treat the industry as a business.

This shift to business logic has created ways to operate more efficiently to decrease health care costs while continuing to maintain quality care to patients and clients. Case managers must apply good business logic to quality treatment and compassion throughout the continuum of care.

To understand the business of health care, it is essential to explore some of the ways that the health care industry acquires its earnings.

For example, many of the health care settings receive their earnings mostly from private insurance, government insurance (Medicare, Medicaid, Medi-Cal, federal employees), military insurance, and private pay. These health care settings include hospitals, sub-acute health care facilities, skilled nursing facilities, home health agencies, ambulatory care clinics, acute psychiatric facilities, hospices, community clinics, school systems, and medical home models.

Acute rehabilitation facilities get earnings from Worker's Compensation as well as the other categories mentioned.

Insurance companies receive their earnings from premiums that are submitted by businesses and corporations who pay for employee's health care coverage. They also receive premiums from individuals.

School systems receive their earnings mostly from state allocated funds in which a designated annual amount is granted to the school for each chronically ill student. They may also receive some federal funding to manage children with such chronic illnesses as diabetes and asthma.

Centers for Medicare and Medicaid Services (CMS) receive government funding to provide insurance coverage to qualified beneficiaries. Many of the health care institutions receive a large amount of their earnings from servicing the Medicare and/or Medicaid beneficiaries. Some institutions receive between 20 to 60 per cent of their revenue from the federal government. This percentage is expected to increase with the aging population and health care reform.

Medi-Cal (California) is state and federally-funded in California. Med-Cal is similar to Medicaid in other states.

Managed Care Organizations (MCO) and Accountable Care Organizations (ACO) receive earnings mostly from employer groups, private insurance, government insurance (Medicare, Medicaid, Medi-Cal, federal employees), military insurance and private pay.

Excellent case management in health care yields two rewards for these many institutions, businesses, government agencies, organizations and corporations. One of the rewards is the reputation that the entity receives for promoting quality and compassionate care throughout the continuum of care. The second reward is the monetary gain and savings that occur from effectively managing the patients and clients in a cost effective environment.

Applying business logic to case management is essential as the future beckons. However, at the same time that case managers are eyeing the bottom line, they must also be aware of the impact of regulatory agencies on their profession. The next chapter will discuss regulatory organizations.

Learn more about the impact of finances on health care. Read "Containing Health Care Costs" in The Merck Manual (http://www. merckmanuals.com/professional/special_subjects/financial_issues_in_ health_care/containing_health_care_costs.html) along with Overview Of Health Care Financing and Causes Of High Health Care Costs.

CHAPTER FOUR

REGULATORY AGENCIES IMPACT CASE MANAGEMENT

"We have to have some rules and regulations in America, or the world would empty out here."

- Gary Ackerman

Health care is one of the most regulated industries in the nation. There are extensive laws that govern health care to promote safe and efficient quality care as well as to promote the effective use of health care spending.

All health care payments are paid by the use of converting the care provided or the procedures performed into International Classification of Diseases (ICD) codes and Current Procedural Treatment Codes (CPT codes). These codes are entered into the claim form for payment to the provider of service.

This chapter will focus on such regulatory agencies as Medicare, Medi-Cal, Medicaid, and others. Case managers must be knowledgeable about these regulations to understand how the financial cycle works. It will also explain how the money is cycled through the health system.

Case managers must start by becoming knowledgeable about Medicare. Medicare was created in 1965 and was intended to provide medical coverage to people over 65 years of age. Medicare now also provides medical coverage for people younger than 65 if they become permanently disabled. The beneficiary or their spouse must have paid into Medicare during their working history prior to retirement or prior to them becoming disabled in order to be eligible for Medicare benefits. Beneficiaries have to apply for Medicare insurance either when they are approaching 65 years of age or when they become permanently disabled.

Medicare was created under title XVIII of the Social Security Act. Today Medicare insures around forty million people in the United States and is the largest insurer in the country.

Medicare Part A covers hospital costs, skilled nursing facilities (SNF) and some home health services. Medicare Part B is a supplemental insurance and covers outpatient and physician costs.

The criteria and guidelines that are used by Medicare drive the commercial insurance industry to adopt the same or similar criteria and guidelines to determine insurance payments in the private sector. Medicare usually pays either all or a portion of the bill when health care resources are used for patients who are Medicare beneficiaries and when the services provided meet the criteria for payment.

To obtain Medicare coverage prior to 65 years of age, the patient must be permanently disabled for two years. In certain diagnosis, permanent disability is declared earlier. For example, the patient has to only wait three months to be eligible for Medicare if he/she has end stage renal disease and is on hemodialysis treatments. The patient must apply for Medicare coverage when they are deemed eligible.

A patient may still work past 65 and be eligible for Medicare insurance at age 65. Patients are encouraged to apply for Medicare about three months before their 65th birthday to have benefits start on time.

Medicare Part B is a supplemental insurance and requires the beneficiary to pay monthly premiums. Patients who have only Part B insurance should have another insurance to cover acute hospitalizations. Medicare is a federal program and individuals are eligible due to work history and retirement eligibility. Medicare benefits are the same for individuals nationwide.

Case managers should be aware that CCH Incorporated publishes an annual guide with updates titled "Medicare Explained." This practical guide is an asset for case managers to help them understand the detailed Medicare regulations. A copy may be obtained by calling 1-800-248-3248, or online at www.health.cch.com.

Medi-Cal (California) is not the same thing as Medicare. It is funded by the State of California with a small amount of federal funding and it is for low income patients and the financially indigent.

Medicaid (CMS) is a federally funded insurance for low income and medically indigent people in other states. The federal government funds Medicaid but allows each state to determine eligibility and benefits, state by state. Therefore, case managers must be aware that benefits under Medicaid may vary from state to state.

Commercial insurance is the same thing as private insurance. For the most part, private insurance companies use the guidelines set up by Medicare to determine expectations and payment determinations.

Another health care regulatory oversight body is The Joint Commission (Accreditation). This is an independent organization that grants facilities a certification for quality care as outlined by the guidelines set by The Joint Commission. Accreditation is mostly in acute hospitals. Medicare (CMS) reimburses payments to acute care facilities that are accredited by The Joint Commission.

The Certified Accreditation for Rehabilitation Facilities (Accreditation) is a certification of facilities that are designated as rehabilitation centers where patients are able to undergo intensive activity to return to their maximum function. Those facilities are deemed to provide high quality standards as outlined in the certification standards.

How do all the health care organizations get paid?

For Medicare (CMS), Medi-Cal (California), Medicaid (CMS), insurance companies, Workers Compensation and Fee for Service, claims need to be filed with appropriate documentation and clinical coding to include ICD and CPT codes.

For Diagnosis Related Group Assignment (DRGs), documentation must include a list of diagnoses that are numbered and assigned a projected length of stay in the acute care hospital. DRGs were created in the early 1980s and each DRG will be given a certain amount of reimbursement dollars. If the provider managers the length of stay within the estimated days, the provider receives money whereas there is the potential to lose money if the length of stay exceeds the amount assigned by the DRG number grouping.

For Perspective Payment System (PPS), the provider is paid a set amount of dollars to manage the patient's care.

The importance of proper documentation throughout the process of care coordination cannot be over-stressed. Medical coders review medical records to apply the appropriate ICD and CPT codes as well as the appropriate DRG assignments. If the documentation is not adequate, the reimbursement from CMS or private insurance to the health care facility will be affected. Documentation will be dealt with in more detail in the next chapter.

Learn more about the International Classification of Diseases (ICD) by visiting the World Health Organization site: http://www.who. int/classifications/icd/en/. There are downloads and full explanations available. More information is also available about Current Procedural Treatment Codes, the numbers a doctor places on insurance forms to describe the services he or she performed. These are published annually by the American Medical Association in CPT codes (there are several editions) and available at the AMA Bookstore: https://catalog.ama-assn. org/Catalog/home.jsp. The book is also available in medical libraries. The CPT codes are also available free for non-commercial use through AMA's CPT page: http://www.ama-assn.org/ama/pub/physician-resources/ solutions-managing-your-practice/coding-billing-insurance/cpt.page.

CHAPTER FIVE

DOCUMENTATION CHALLENGES

"I'm a hoarder. For me, documentation has always been key, and I've kept everything from my past."

- Diane Keaton

Regardless of what setting or process you encounter along the continuum of care, the health care adage that "If it wasn't documented, it wasn't done," applies.

It is true for the process of keeping the patient moving from one appropriate setting to the next. It is especially true in the reimbursement world for health care. If diagnoses, treatment, and services are not documented in the medical record, the health care facility will not be paid.

This issue has become so important that in recent years a new position called a clinical documentation specialist has been created in many health care organizations. The role of the clinical documentation specialist is to review medical records to ensure the provider has adequately documented in the medical records to maximize reimbursement dollars.

In facilities where the organization is fortunate enough to have a clinical documentation specialist, the person will work either directly or indirectly with the case management department.

Reporting structure varies with each organization. The clinical documentation specialist will monitor documentation in the medical record to ensure that the organization is coding and billing insurance companies appropriately for services provided. This person may also be a liaison for the recovery audit coordinator (RAC) in the organization.

This position is mostly held by nurses but could be held by other health care workers who are knowledgeable about the documentation rules.

Documentation is one of the case manager's roles as well. They must document what they know about each patient's case. This documentation provides information to the health care team about the plan of care and allows for communication about any patient or family dynamic.

To be effective, the case manager's documentation must be accurate and concise. Writing should be neat and legible. The case manager must document information regarding transfers, potential problems, patient's non-compliance, and any contacts for staff awareness.

Case management documentation should tell the patient's story from admission to discharge. This detailed information should be communicated to everyone involved with the planned next steps of the patient's health care.

At all levels of documentation, the introduction of the electronic health record (EHR) in health care is clearly one of the most integrated functions to come along in the health care industry in the 21st century. The seamless movement of data speeds up the process for medical treatments, medical transactions, and reduces medical errors. The electronic health record makes data readily available when it is needed.

Most importantly, the EHR appears to improve the quality of care without increasing the cost of care. Sharing of valuable patient information through EHR allows for better treatment coordination in a timely manner.

While a key role in documentation is preparing and providing written evidence of treatments for patients, an accompanying skill is needed. The skill is to develop an open attitude about the process. A case manager must be amenable to receiving and sharing information about the patient and the plan of care, not only for the short term but also for the long term.

It is only through the process of getting and giving information that achievable goals can be established with the patient, the family, and the multidisciplinary health care team.

The case manager may take the center role of leading the entire group into productive discharge planning. It is the case manager who will ensure that the patient and family know the direction in which the team is trying to move them. The patient and family should be allowed to verbalize their understanding about the care plan.

Documenting and sharing information is also vital in achieving an efficient discharge outcome. The sooner the case manager begins to dialogue with the patient, family and health care team, the higher the likelihood of a favorable outcome. If the health care team has advance knowledge of a patient's need for care coordination, as in the event of an elective procedure, for example, the process can be accomplished in a transparent manner.

Case managers will also come across insurance companies, managed care organizations, health plans, and health maintenance organizations that require patients to get pre approval for certain medical visits, treatments, procedures, and hospitalizations before proceeding.

The case manager may be the person designated to discuss the authorizations with the payer source. In the event that the case manager obtains authorization for payment, he or she must have all the details about the patient and know specifically what services is requested and why. To obtain this information, the case manager will need to have a dialogue with the care provider.

If an authorization is not obtained as required by the payer, the claim may be denied when it is submitted for payment. This causes the patient to pay out of pocket for care or the provider may have to take a loss for the service provided.

Case managers may not win every battle, but the more focused they are on insisting on excellent documentation and taking the time to understand it thoroughly, the better results they will be able to achieve for their patients. Sometimes their task will be smooth and sometimes harder. Even when all the records are in order and the case manager knows all aspects of the case, it can suddenly become difficult because of unanticipated changes. In the next chapter, some of the skills to handle tough situations will be discussed.

The Association of Clinical Documentation Improvement Specialists is a community in which CDI professionals share strategies for successful documentation improvement programs and achieve professional growth. Their website (http://www.hcpro.com/acdis/) offers a relevant blog on documentation and the association itself offers a number of e-learning programs for documentation improvement. The list of courses currently available in the ACDIS library is available at: http://www.hcpro.com/acdis/intralearn.cfm.

CHAPTER SIX

COLLABORATION WITH
DIFFICULT PEOPLE

"I think of difficult people as my teacher instead of my enemy."

- Author Unknown

The case manager's work with patients and their families can be very challenging at times. There is no "one size fits all" solution to dealing with difficulties, but professionalism, compassion and excellent communication skills can go a long way to solving the problems.

Being knowledgeable about the patient's case and able to empathize with the patients and their families is also important. Most patients and their families want to be kept abreast of the situation and changes in condition. Keeping them updated on all situations is another key role that the case manager can fill.

At times patients and families are labeled as difficult to deal with when in actuality, the difficult behavior may be a coping mechanism for fear and frustration because someone on the health care team has not listened or taken the time to fully understand the family dynamics.

No one family has the same issues as another. The case manager may be the person who is in a position to diffuse some of their fear and frustration.

The universal need that patients and families have during a period of illness is hope. The case manager can act as a liaison between the family and the health care team. The case manager can allow the family to vent and ask questions and then educate them on the crisis situation.

Case managers can help families to be empowered to make decisions and help them to cope. The case manager should talk with patients and family members frequently, if needed, to prevent fear, anger, and anxiety. The difficult family in many situations will become more cooperative when they know that they are being heard, when they know that they matter and when they sense that their concerns are being answered honestly.

From time to time, the case manager may also have the experience of dealing with difficult doctors. As the saying goes, doctors are human too. They do not escape the problems that everyone encounters in their careers or their personal lives. However, in the health care setting, the case manager is expected to be respected as one of the critical people to assist with care coordination, discharge planning, and care along the care continuum.

There are things case managers can do to increase effective communications with doctors. These include having a good overview of what is going on with each patient on his/her caseload before beginning the conversation with a doctor about moving the patient to the next level of care.

Case managers are not expected to have personal knowledge of each and every detail of a disease process. However, they should have resources, nursing handbooks, or medical reference textbooks on the desk and on line so that they can quickly reference the disease, review the prognosis, and acquire some idea about what the plan of care should be for the current stage of the patient's illness.

The case manager should be able to confidently have a conversation with the physician about the next steps that may be available for the patient from a case manager's perspective. It is necessary to be careful to honor the physician's role and not to appear as if the case manager is trying to replace the physician's plan of care and "practice medicine."

Remember that some physicians believe that many case managers do not have a clear picture of what is going on with the patient's disease process. They sometimes think that the case manager's primary concern is "when will this patient be discharged?"

In cases like these, it is possible that the case manager has not yet established a mutual relationship with the physician. The nurse case manager could be experiencing some discomfort in communicating with a particular physician, especially if that doctor has a reputation of hesitating to move patients to the appropriate level of care.

An ideal way to handle this situation is for the case manager to be able to quickly articulate their knowledge of the case to the physician and to recommend alternate resources that could be safe and appropriate at the next level.

Getting right to the point is another excellent skill for the case manager to develop. Physicians want case managers to be knowledgeable about the patient's plan of care, but they also want the case manager to be able to keep their conversation brief as a sign of respect for the physician's busy schedule. Yet some nurses and case managers have a tendency to provide a long narrative for each situation before getting to the point. The physicians want the case manager to get to the point quickly.

An excellent method for case managers to adopt is called SBAR, which means to talk to the physician in succinct terms about Situation, Background, Assessment and Recommendation for the patient. The conversation will be succinct, but also cover all bases effectively.

As this chapter has already illustrated, case managers are asked to communicate with a variety of people who have different degrees of understanding of the health care process. They need to candidly discuss the plan of care with the multidisciplinary team, the patient, the family, internal and external staff, and the people who are following the patient in the community.

Even more challenging, each person wants to be communicated with on their level, whether they are chief executive officers, patients, senior leaders, physicians, families or community liaisons.

Additionally, the case manager will have to use two levels of language. When communicating with the professional group, the case managers will problem solve with the group using professional terminology. On the other hand, the problem solving with the family will be discussed using the language of laypeople.

Add to these challenges the reality that the case manager must also be able to identify diverse cultural needs, and it becomes clear why the professional case manager should invest considerable time and effort in developing excellent communication skills.

It is also worth mentioning how important it is that the case manager who has to handle all these difficulties should be aware that they must always "look the part" if they are to get past first base with those who would challenge them. Case managers are professionals and the attire they select during working hours should reflect a professional unity.

Business casual is appropriate. In certain environments such as the hospital setting, many case managers may be required to wear a white lab coat over their casual business dress. In other settings and in the community environment, business casual is acceptable without a lab coat.

The case manager must exhibit professional judgment of integrity to promote great patient care. Appearance can have a big impact on how one sees himself/herself and how many who are in contact with the case manager view them.

In the next chapter we will look at a yet another challenging area for the case manager, and that is handling cases involving children.

Read more about techniques for handling difficult people. Two articles to start with are "Dealing with Difficult People" by Dr. Nando Pelusi on the Psychology Today website: http://www.psychologytoday.com/ articles/200609/dealing-difficult-people and Tips On Managing Difficult People on the Harvard Business Review site: http://hbr.org/web/ management-tip/tips-on-managing-difficult-people. Armed with these techniques, consider one of the most difficult clients, physicians or families you have handled in the last week and think about ways you might have handled the situation more effectively. Start your own file of techniques that work well for you.

CHAPTER SEVEN

CARE COORDINATION IN THE PEDIATRIC POPULATION

"We worry about what a child will become tomorrow, yet we forget that he is someone today."

- Stacia Tauscher

The case management of children is very different from case managing adults. Unlike adult case management, the case management of children can have a multitude of factors surrounding the children, their families and their living environments.

Pediatric case management can span from simple, short lived illnesses or can expand into the management of more complex chronic and long term developmentally challenged cases.

Children in the acute care setting may have short length of stays (LOS) when they are admitted for an episodic event such as an elective surgery or for a short term illness such as bronchitis. The pediatric case manager must involve a multidisciplinary team to determine the plan of care. The parents/family must be included in the plan of care decisions.

Many of the chronically managed pediatric cases will involve local, state and federal governance.

Case managers who work with the pediatric population must deal with the child, their family, primary care physicians, specialty physicians, and other health care team members. The case manager must also be able to manage his or her emotions as it relates to the child's illness or special needs.

Case management models for children should integrate the acute and chronic plans of care to ensure that the child, the family, and the primary care physician are fully engaged and involved in the decision making, while making sure that it is centered on the child, the family dynamics, and the resources in the community that will support the patient.

The pediatric case manager must be fully aware of the different developmental stages that children go through and be able to recognize what stage the assigned patient is at and realize when the transition from one stage to the next is beginning. This is especially important when the child is being case managed long term due to a chronic illness or developmental disability.

Pediatric case management can consume large amounts of time and resources. In developmentally disabled children, the federal requirement is that they undergo continuing disability reviews about every three years. Once the child reaches 18 years of age, it is required that he or she have their disability re-evaluated.

Pediatric case managers must understand various insurance coverage policies. The child may have a private insurance coverage through the parent's insurance coverage, but this does not always mean that the patient is not eligible for other local, state, and/or federal public funding programs.

The Social Security Act covers Children with Special Health Care Needs (CSHCN). Although CSHCN is funded by a combination of federal, state and local funds, each program is administered by the county or state and the funding is governed by Title V of the Social Security administration.

Several publicly funded programs that were developed to help underserved children are The State Children's Health Insurance Program (SCHIP), the Department of Developmental Disabilities, and Special Supplement Nutrition Program for Women, Infants, and Children (WIC).

This book provides a basic overview of pediatric case management. Case managers who are interested in engaging in this field as a specialty are encouraged to attend classes that are tailored to children and their dynamic management models.

For case managers interested in specializing in pediatric case management, consult "Pediatric Life Care Planning and Case Management, Second Edition" edited by Susan Riddick-Grisham and Laura Deming (http://www.amazon.com/Pediatric-Life-Planning-Management-Second/dp/1439803587). It is a comprehensive review that goes beyond clinical discussion to include legal and financial aspects, life expectancy data, and assistive technology. Case samples of actual plans related to specific conditions are included.

CHAPTER EIGHT

PROFESSIONAL DEVELOPMENT FOR THE CASE MANAGER

"Education is not piling on of learning, information, data, facts, skills, or abilities—that's training or instruction—but is rather making visible what is hidden as a seed."

- Thomas Moore

To be an effective case manager, the health care worker will spend considerable time learning about the various settings along the health care continuum. The awareness of rules and regulations governing insurance programs and local, state and federal guidelines are key to being an effective case manager.

All of this education will help to make them capable, but to excel in this role case managers must hone another set of skills, many of which they have already learned and are hidden deep inside of them. Now will be the time to summon them to the surface.

For example, the ability to collaborate is crucial. Webster Dictionary defines "collaboration" as the ability to work jointly with others toward a common goal.

In health care case management, the case manager is at the center of the collaborative process. He/she must be involved in the communication with the provider and the multidisciplinary team to determine the plan of care. The case manager, along with the provider, must be pivotal in communicating this plan to the patient, the family, and any other entity along the planned continuum of care.

The collaborative process will involve staff internal to the patient's current setting and can extend externally to other settings such as skilled rehabilitation, for example.

Additionally, the case manager will be responsible for communicating with authorized personnel at insurance companies and managed health care organizations to share the care plan, expected outcome, and patient's discharge disposition.

Just as important as the ability to collaborate for case managers is the ability to utilize critical thinking skills. This means to use careful judgment in making decisions while thinking about situations in a global scope.

The health care case manager must be able to visualize a global view of what is and what could be possible. He/she must be able to think innovatively because there will not be any two case management situations that will be the same.

Even if the patient returns to the same setting in the future for treatment, the plan of care may not always be the same. The case manager may be the person who has to recommend alternative arrangements which may seem unrealistic to the multidisciplinary team, the patient, and the family. Some of the alternatives may even seem farfetched to the case manager himself/herself. However, the case manager is the one person who can pull the pieces of the resource puzzle to fit together in the end somehow. The case manager must always be open to new possibilities.

Hand in hand with collaboration and critical thinking goes conflict resolution skills. The case manager will come into contact with people on a regular basis in which conflict will be a large part of the case management process. The case manager will need to mediate various situations involving the multidisciplinary team, the patient, and the family.

The first type of conflict may be that with the professional staff. When roles and job descriptions are not defined to the team, there is a degree of assumptions from all parties. It is necessary for the case manager to clarify with his/her manager regarding the expectations of the position.

Additionally, it is essential that the administration and other team members understand the case manager's role. Therefore, the role clarification decreases the miscommunication, role overlap and diffuses perceptions.

The second type of conflict for the case manager is that of handling the plan of care with the patient and the family members. This type of conflict will repeat itself over and over in case management. There is not any one situation that presents itself in the same manner. The case manager must be the mediator who eventually mediates with an acceptable outcome.

Conflict exists in every job situation as well as personal relationships. The effective case manager will recognize the importance of conflict resolution skills and seek out further training by attending courses, engaging in reading about this subject, and discussing conflict resolution with more experienced case managers.

Conflict is inevitable when there is more than one person in any situation. Prepare for conflict and plan you next mediation strategies.

When collaboration and conflict are part of your daily routine, there exists opportunities for stress to enter the equation. In the next chapter we will look at stress in the case manager's position and ways to manager a challenging case load.

The nature of health management is constantly changing and evolving. As a result, it is vital to stay abreast with change through continuing education and reading. The book "Case Management: An Introduction to Concepts and Skills," Third Edition by Arthur J. Frankel (University of North Carolina, Wilmington) and Sheldon R. Gelman (Yeshiva University)(http://lyceumbooks.com/casemgt3ed.htm) is attentive to the evolving needs of a variety of populations and it now contains a new section on working with members of the military and their families.

CHAPTER NINE

STRESS MANAGEMENT FOR THE CASE MANAGER

"It's not stress that kills us, it is our reaction to it."

- Hans Selye

The position of case manager requires a great deal of time and if the case manager is not organized, the workload can become stressful and frustration sets in until it becomes "burn out."

It is crucial to learn how to prioritize and learn how to walk away from a situation that does not command immediate attention. If it can be done tomorrow, it may have to wait.

Stress can also be reduced by anticipating demands and questions that will come at the case manager from all directions. For example, know what it is you need before you telephone the insurance company. Time will not be wasted with unnecessary conversation or the need to make a second call.

Learn to delegate tasks to other team members. It is not necessary for the case manager to do everything. Case managers need to accept that others can do work correctly, and that they don't have to do everything themselves. Delegate.

Case managers individual caseload assignments will depend on many variables and the senior leadership's commitment to staff according to acuity levels.

Among some of the variables to consider when assigning caseloads are the types of patients, payer demands for authorizations, principal diagnosis, chronic illness cases, and travel distances between cases.

There are many other variables to consider. For example, the pediatric caseload will vary depending on the setting. In the hospital, the assigned cases may be similar to the adult acute caseload of 15, 20, or 25. In the community setting the caseload will be higher. If there are children with special needs and disabilities, the caseload assignment should take into consideration the large amount of time that it takes to work with this special needs population.

The caseload for the behavioral health case manager varies depending on the intensity of the patients. Patients may be case managed in an intense inpatient program or they may be on maintenance therapy in the community.

The caseload for a home health case manager ranges from 30-60 lives depending on the severity of illness. The caseload for ambulatory care settings could range anywhere from 50-100 or more cases depending on the type of patients that are assigned to the case worker. In the wellness clinic, where most patients are relatively healthy, a caseworker may handle a higher volume due to infrequent encounters.

The caseload for the chronic disease case manager may range from 30 to 60 depending on the extent of the acuity of the patients who make up this caseload.

The ideal caseload for a case manager in acute care settings ranges from 15-25 patients. However, the reality of an assignment in the acute setting can routinely be 25-30. When the acute care assignment is over 25, it is beginning to be a heavy caseload. The goal of cost effective management of the patients' cases could be ineffective at this level.

The skilled nursing case manager caseload could be somewhat higher than that of the acute care case manager but less than the assigned caseload for the community case manager. The rehabilitation case manager's caseload will depend on the type of facility and the severity of illness of the patients. It will most likely be similar to that of the skilled nursing case manager.

The average caseload for the workers compensation case manager will depend on many factors such as the severity of the cases and whether they are short-term, long-term, or catastrophic cases. The case worker may have a mix of the various types of cases.

Case managers in the community clinics tend to have large caseloads. For the school nurse, the caseload also varies depending on whether the case manager is assigned to one school or multiple school sites. Within the Department of Justice, the caseload varies depending on the number of sites that are assigned to a caseworker.

Balancing the case manager's workload is a continuously moving target that must be met with a supportive team approach. The team must also consider caseload adjustments based on such factors as family dynamics, the time it takes to gather and analyze data to make appropriate decisions based on utilization, case management, and quality improvement for each case that is being handled.

The role of a case manager can be very stressful. The health care case manager's role will become more important, more necessary, and more demanding with health care reform and with the aging population.

Each case manager must decide on what it is outside of work that gives them joy. They must engage in whatever it is that makes them happy, be it small or large. Case managers deserve to take care of their needs.

It is important for case managers to remind themselves that they are needed in the health care field. Burn out in this role is not the destiny for them. To avoid it, case managers need to take needed time away from work. They must use their vacation time, whether it is one day or one month, to revitalize themselves.

Case managers need to spend time with important people in their lives. Sometimes they may need to leave work early to treat themselves to ice cream, take in a movie, meet a friend, or join a support group that will help to create a stress free life balance.

Consider attending classes on issues related to case management to keep current with the profession. Case managers who keep current with their roles experience less stress in their practice. Sometimes it also helps to attend a seminar on time management and act on the skills it provides. It is important for case managers to manage their time effectively. The efficient case manager learns to plan ahead, make lists, and use time management skills.

If a case manager suddenly realizes that the job is completely draining him/her, they must re-evaluate the position and determine if it is time to move to the next career stage. It may be time for a resume update.

It is vital for case managers to meet the demands of others to purposely take a time out for self care to stay healthy. The case manager must embrace a work life balance.

Take time out for a self-examination. How well are you achieving work life balance? Take stock regularly to ensure your daily activities match your personal goals. Read the newest literature on dealing with work/life stress. For further reading, consult "Tweak It: Make What Matters To You Happen Every Day" by thought leader Cali Williams Yost. (http://www. amazon.ca/Tweak-Matters-Happen-Every-ebook/dp/B007ZFIPLY/ref=sr _1_2?s=books&ie=UTF8&qid=1362429961&sr=1-2)

CHAPTER TEN

DENIAL OF SERVICES

*"Refusal to believe until proof is given is a rational position;
denial of all outside of our own limited experience is absurd.*

- Annie Besant

Case managers must be aware of the procedures and processes to follow when a service, durable medical equipment, or a submitted claim is not approved by the payer source / insurance company.

Generally the service provider is a hospital, a rehabilitation facility, or a clinic.

In the hospital, the attending physician and the utilization / case management department must be in agreement to issue the letter to the patient or their family.

Documentation of denials must be clearly notated in the records.

Medicare and some private insurance firms have a standard method for the denial process. Case managers must review the standard criteria for denial of services and ensure that they have followed the necessary steps to provide the service denial.

Patients and institutions can appeal decisions to deny services or denial of claims payments. With adequate and justifiable documentation of medical necessity for services, the denial may be overturned in favor of the patient and/or the institution.

Some of the reasons services may be denied are that they were provided at the wrong level of care, they are not covered by the insurance/health plan, the provider had to obtain prior authorization and did not, the admission to a hospital was not necessary for diagnosis, and the claim was not submitted in a timely fashion for payment. Lack of documentation to justify the services is another reason for denial.

In times such as these, and in many others, the case manager may find themselves adding to their role the job of patient advocate. This is defined as being the support for patients and families who are unable to speak for themselves or are unable to recognize what steps to take next.

As the case manager, it is expected that this role would prepare the patient and the family for the maximum chance to sustain the best possible experience and the best patient outcome at the end of the continuum of care.

As nurses transition from the bedside into the field of case management, and as social workers or other health care workers take on the role of case management, they must remember this role. They must keep it in their minds even with the intent to be cost effective and time sensitive in managing the plan of care along the continuum. Always advocate for the patient.

The role of advocating for the patient to have the desired quality of care must continue to be the primary focus. The case manager is the advocate and the gatekeeper.

Standing firm to speak for the patient and be a patient advocate in spite of the obstacles may not always be the popular thing to do, but it will always be the right thing to do. Effective case managers must remember to act on the right thing.

Consider how patient advocacy fits into your role as a case manager. Download the free publication, "Patient Advocacy for Health Care Quality, Strategies for Achieving Patient-Centered Care" from Jones and Bartlett Publishers of Sudbury, Mass. Written by Jo Anne L. Earp, ScD, professor and chair of Health Behavior and Health Education at the University of North Carolina at Chapel Hill, Elizabeth A. French, MA, a lecturer in that same department, and Melissa B. Gilkey, MPH, Johns

Hopkins Bloomberg School of Public Health, Baltimore, the book creates thought-provoking strategies for all health providers to consider.

(http://www.jblearning.com/samples/0763749613/49613_fm.pdf)

Read "The Patient Advocate's Handbook: 300 Questions and Answers to Help You Care for Your Loved One at the Hospital and at Home" by James Thomas Williams. This patient advocate book discussed common situations created by illness and recovery to offer relevant information when it is needed. It illustrates how an advocate can have a more effective experience.

(http://www.amazon.com/Patient-Advocates-Handbook-Questions-Hospital/dp/0984282505)

CHAPTER ELEVEN

ESSENTIAL LEADERSHIP FOR CASE MANAGERS

"A genuine leader is not a searcher for consensus but a molder of consensus."

- Martin Luther King, Jr.

Case managers are leaders in their field. They have to understand the business of health care and ensure efficient use of resources.

In practical terms, this means they must stay current with the latest developments in the delivery and development of efficient health care services.

A vast amount of resources exist for case management. One can search for just about any topic on the Internet and find instant answers to questions.

Case managers are also advised to select user friendly textbooks, magazines, articles, and websites to keep up to date on their profession. It is also good practice to regularly attend seminars and conferences in the field of case management.

Every case manager should also have a personal resource library that includes at minimum a list of community references, websites for patient and family references, professional colleagues, local networks, and resources for specialty areas that they may not have expertise in, but may on occasion be assigned to case manage.

As case managers gain experience, they should also become a resource for new case managers.

Each case manager should also have their own toolkit to help in performing the case management role effectively. The toolkit should include the tools that make the day-to-day operations go smoother.

Part of the toolkit will include some type of organization system for assignments such as an agenda, binder, or laptop computer notes.

Other tools include the guidelines used to determine medical necessity.

When case managers find themselves having to work in a specialty for which they have no previous experience, it is essential to take the time to research the cases so that an informed and intelligent dialogue can be held with the patient, the family, and the health care team.

The first twelve to twenty-four months of working as a case manager is sufficient time for a person to determine if they will enjoy this career choice. The first year is more of an introduction to this area of health care.

At the three year point, case managers should be determining if they would like to become certified. They now have the experience and skills to fully understand the position and are now eligible to apply for the certification examination.

At five years into the case management role, practitioners should be at a space where they are considered somewhat of an expert in the area. This is a great time for case managers to consider mentoring other nurses, social workers, and health care professionals into becoming case managers.

Case managers are encouraged to set realistic career goals and to set aside moments to reflect on the direction and desire of their chosen profession.

After three to five years, case managers may want to consider a leadership role in their area.

Take some time to consider how you can develop your leadership skills and apply them to your work as a case manager. To read more about this subject, consult "Leadership in Health Care," by Jill Barr and Lesley Dowding. (http://www.amazon.com/Leadership-Health-Care-Jill-Barr/ dp/1412920671). This publication addresses the need for leading skilled and evidence based care within the context of a performance measured health service. It offers support to those training to be health care professionals by identifying the breadth of leadership theory that they can apply to their own practice.

CHAPTER TWELVE

CASE MANAGEMENT
CERTIFICATION

"You are educated. Your certification is in your degree. You may think of it as the ticket to the good life. Let me ask you to think of an alternative. Think of it as your ticket to change the world."

- Tom Brokaw

Certification For Individuals: ACMA, CMSA

Many types of case management certification certificates exist to validate that a person has the expertise and knowledge to practice at the specified level of their professional credentialing.

The two most popular case management certifications are granted by the Case Management Society of America (CMSA) and the American Case Management Association (ACMA).

The Case Management Association of America is one of the major organizations that certify professional individuals to be credentialed as case managers. The professional standards of practice for case managers were created by CMSA in 1993.

It is estimated that 30,000 case managers have taken the exam and are certified case managers (CCM).

The certified case manager's examination focuses on six core areas of case management: case management concepts, case management principles, psychosocial and support systems, health care delivery, health care reimbursement, and vocational concepts and strategies.

Becoming a certified case manager is a voluntary credential but more and more case management positions prefer certifications to meet the job requirement specifications.

The case manager goes through an application process to write the certification exams and must have the minimum years of experience as required by the testing organization. Most applications require a minimum of two years of on the job experience before taking the examination.

The American Case Management Association (ACMA) focuses on collaborative case management in the hospital/health care organization for patients, nurses, social workers, physicians, caregivers, and the community. Case managers can become certified by taking the examination for the ACMA.

Certification sets the individual case manager apart from others and is considered to be a preference when applying for a case management position.

Certifications For Organizations: URAC

Case Management Accreditation
And Certification Program Overview

URAC is the only accreditation organization offering standards that specifically address the rapidly evolving field of case management for organizations.

URAC has accredited hundreds of organizations that provide all types of case management services, in both health and workers' compensation settings, helping ensure that their case management offerings are of the highest quality. URAC designed the standards to fit organizations that provide telephonic or onsite case management services in conjunction with a privately or publicly funded benefits program across settings and specialties. Accreditation or certification is available depending on the type of organization and services being offered.

The URAC standards cover several critical operational categories for any quality case management program including staff structure and organization, staff management and development, information management, quality improvement, oversight of delegated functions, organizational ethics and complaints.

URAC works directly with organizations to establish their baseline operational level at the beginning of the review process. Written policies and procedures that include a definition of case management, the types of consumers served, the delivery model for case management services and case management staff qualifications are reviewed.

According to the business development team at URAC, guidelines for reasonable caseload and sufficient personnel to provide services to consumers are established. Policies requiring licensed physicians be available for consultations with case managers are put in place, as well as ensuring continuing education meeting nationally recognized standards is available for all case managers.

The URAC Case Management Accreditation Standards, which are built on the Core Accreditation Standards, enable organizations to successfully train case managers, identify individuals for case management, manage and conduct case management activities in an efficient and professional manner, promote the autonomy of consumer and family decision making, maintain confidentiality and delegate responsibility.

Contact URAC to join the group of Case Management Accredited and Certified companies. Call (202) 216-9010 for more information. (http://www.urac.org/).

Consider your career choices in the field of case management. On the website of the Case Management Society of America (http://www.cmsa. org/) you will find an industry director. On the website of the American Case Management Association (http://www.acmaweb.org/), you will find Career Link, a way of connecting yourself to employment opportunities.

CHAPTER THIRTEEN

INTERDEPENDENCE OF CEOS, PROVIDERS, AND CASE MANAGERS

"Change is the law of life. And those who look only to the past or present are certain to miss the future."

- John F. Kennedy

What does full implementation of the Affordable Health Care Act mean to health care leaders? How will the health care paradigm shift for the health care case manager? How will senior leadership handle the demand for case managers?

The chief executive officer (CEO) is responsible for the bottom line in health care organizations, but the buck stops with case management.

Over the next three to five years, the health care environment will experience chaos which will require major shifts in thought, operations, and care management. As the industry enters unpaved healthcare markets, it is impossible to fathom all of the required shifts. Case management may become the saving face for health care spending provided case managers are trained and educated to be great clinicians with savvy strategic thinking to align quality patient care with cost savings.

Health care case managers—nurses, social workers, health care professionals—must shift their thinking into a logical business manner. The health care industry will present tremendous demand for case managers to manage patients across all levels of care. Equally expected is the supply deficit of well trained case managers to meet the demand. In business school they call this the economics of supply and demand. When the supply is plentiful, services seem not as valuable because there are too many workers. When the demand is high, the value of service costs more because there are simply not enough workers.

For a short period, health care case managers will have the power to optimize working conditions due to the lack of well trained health care case managers to meet market demands.

Repetition of the recent health care publications quote is truly fitting of the impending, full implementation of the Affordable Care Act of 2010/ Health Care Report:

"It was the best of times, it was the worst of times, it was the age of wisdom, it was the age of foolishness, it was the epoch of belief, it was the epoch of incredulity, it was the season of light, it was the season of darkness, it was the spring of hope, it was the winter of despair, we had everything before us, we had nothing before us . . ."—Charles Dickens in *A Tale of Two Cities*.

In other words, today we can only predict, without any certainty, the immediate future for health care management. It is an exciting time to be a case manager or to become one. Achieving a spirit of professional collaboration is the best strategy to help provide effective and efficient care for all patients.

The profession of case management and its infiltration into the health care system is growing rapidly and there are no signs that it will go away. In fact, the third annual Health Care Case Management e-survey of 153 health care organizations in 2012 found that ninety percent used case managers. The proportion of case managers working in primary care settings increased from fourteen percent in 2011 to fifty-eight percent in 2012.

Senior leaders in health care facilities are looking at case managers as a means to reduce emergency department visits and hospital admissions as well as improve patient outcomes across the continuum of care.

Organizations will experience a decrease in spending and an increase in return on investment (ROI) if they ensure their case management department is adequately staffed, educated, and committed to keeping updated on the ever changing regulatory environment of care coordination.

Case managers who continue to educate themselves on the rapidly changing world of healthcare will be far ahead of any other professionals in health care. The role of the case manager has been carved out of necessity and competence to help improve the health care crisis and to reduce spending. Case managers must educate the health care team about the important role that they play on the team. The chief executive officers, providers, and case managers must realize the buck stops with case management even though the CEO is responsible for the bottom line.

Meanwhile, there is an important message to send to all health care chief executive officers, senior health care leaders and providers:

The case management department, the case managers, the transitional care coordinators, the embedded case managers, and the community case managers are the team of people who are key to managing the length of stay, preventing unnecessary admissions, reducing readmissions, and ensuring that patients remain compliant with the plan of care along the continuum.

By effectively managing patient flow, the organization's shrinking reimbursements are brought in line to maintain financial stability. When the case management staff is supported by senior leadership to be adequately educated, adequately resourced and highly recognized for their contributions to the bottom line, the tipping point occurs. The tipping point can either save and/or create millions of dollars for the organization.

Think about the effectiveness of collaboration between physicians, senior leadership, and case workers and how it can have a positive impact on the patient. Make a list of the positive benefits achieved when health care facilities employ case managers.

For a case in point, read:

http://www.dorlandhealth.com/case_management/cip_magazine/ Case-Manager-and-Physician-Collaboration-Building-Outcome-Based- Relationships_2061.html

CHAPTER FOURTEEN

HEALTH CARE REFORM . . . WHAT NOW?

"After a century of striving, after a year of debate, after a historic vote, health care reform is no longer an unmet promise. It is the law of the land."

- US President Barack Obama

Since March 23, 2010 when United States President Barack Obama signed the Patient Protection and Affordable Care Act, comprehensive health reforms came into reality and the role of the case manager became even more vital. The purpose of health care reform is to expand health care coverage, control health care costs, and improve the health care delivery systems in the United States of America.

Its overall approach will require most United States citizens and legal residents to have health insurance. Medicaid (Medi-Cal in California) is expanded for those who are considered to be at the federal poverty level. (The poverty level for a family of three in 2009 was $18,310.)

Individual mandate requires U.S. citizens and legal residents to have qualifying health coverage. Those without coverage will pay an individual annual penalty of $695 per year or up to three times that amount ($2,085) for family coverage.

This penalty will be phased in over a three year period starting in 2014 through 2016. Beginning after 2016, the penalty will be increased annually based on the cost of living adjustment.

Exemptions from this penalty will be granted for financial hardship, religious objections, American Indians, those without coverage for less than three months, undocumented immigrants, incarcerated individuals, and those with incomes below the tax filing threshold. The penalty payments will most likely be paid during the individual's annual tax filing.

Medicaid benefits will be expanded to all non-Medicare eligible individuals under age 65 (children, pregnant women, parents, and adults without dependent children) with incomes based on an adjusted federal poverty level income.

The future for the Children's Health Insurance Program (CHIP) changes too. States are required to maintain current income eligibility levels for children in Medicaid and the CHIP program.

As case managers look to their future, they will see a strong picture of their involvement in every health care setting along the continuum of care. There will be challenging times ahead, but also satisfying ones as the profession continues to evolve.

Stay informed about the evolution of health care and the impact of legislative changes on how you work. Make it a point to read and listen to the daily news about health care and participate in discussions to learn the ideas and opinions of others. As a leader in your field, it is important that you stay well informed and aware of changing trends and ideas. Get involved in the professional organizations of case management and become a case manager that will not only make a difference for the patients but will help create and mold the "agents of change" for the profession.

ABOUT THE AUTHOR

Pauline Sanders has been a pioneer in the field of case management theory and practical implementation since 1991. As the President and Program Director for *elite CASE MANAGEMENT*, she is known for her unique passion and ability to train nurses, medical social workers, healthcare workers, and providers to transition into the case management experience with a focus on organizational goals and the patients' well being.

Pauline is a registered nurse who holds a Bachelor's Degree in Health Services Administration from St. Mary's College in Moraga, California, and a Master of Business Administration from the University of Phoenix in Phoenix, Arizona. She is a healthcare leader, consultant, professional speaker, educator, and author. She has more than 25 years experience in Healthcare Quality Management which includes case management, utilization, and discharge planning. She is a certified case manager (CCM) with the Case Management Society of America.

Pauline also has certifications in risk management (CPHRM) from the American Society of Healthcare Risk Management (ASHRM) and legal nurse consulting (LNCC) from the American Association of Legal Nurse Consultants (AALNC).

She is a member of various associations which include the National Association of Professional Women (NAPW), the Women's Speakers Association (WSA), Bay Area Chapter of Nurse Consultants, American Association of Legal Nurse Consultants, American Society of Risk Management, and the Case Management Society of America.

Pauline was recently recognized in Cambridge Who's Who for outstanding professional and personal achievements.

She lives in Northern California and is employed in the Quality Department of a large health and hospital system which is located in San Jose, California.

"I firmly believe that as healthcare workers become trained on the basics of case management and as they grow with the changes in the industry, they will move into the number one position as the most important person on the healthcare team. They will ensure that the circle of needs is connected throughout the continuum of care. The never ending cycle of case management will result in a win-win outcome for healthcare organizations as well as for the patients."—P. Sanders, RN

www.ingramcontent.com/pod-product-compliance
Lightning Source LLC
Chambersburg PA
CBHW022132170526
45157CB00004B/1857